Won Ton and Hissie

January 2016

To dear Clare

with lots of love

Nini xx

Bettina Blume

Hillman Publishing

First Paperback edition printed 2016 in the United Kingdom

Published by:
Hillman Publishing
Email: books@hillmanpublishing.co.uk
Web: www.hillmanpublishing.co.uk

ISBN 978-1-909996-10-6

A Catalogue record for this book is available from the British Library.

Typset in 13pt Garamond by Hillman Publishing

.

Hillman Publishing is an imprint of Coastal Peak Ltd

Dedicated to our cats,
Bignose and Chica

CHAPTER ONE

CAT, MOUSE AND BIRDS

To all appearances, Won Ton was a fortunate cat. Along with his sister, he lived with his owners, Aaron and Rebecca, in a big Georgian house in London filled with treasures from Aaron and Rebecca's travels. It was a beautiful place with an enchanting back garden. Camellias and rhododendrons grew in abundance around the house. There was a rose garden and beyond that a small apple orchard; jasmine grew on the walls and an ancient oak that was over three hundred years old shaded the back lawn. Right at the back of the garden was a fox den that had grown into a warren, helped by the rabbit population from the heath nearby. Sometimes, to their short-lived surprise, curious rabbits found themselves inside the den. There were lots of big rooms in the house with windows reaching from floor to ceiling and massive marble fireplaces. The heart of the house was the kitchen with its big Aga. Its constant warmth made everyone feel wel-

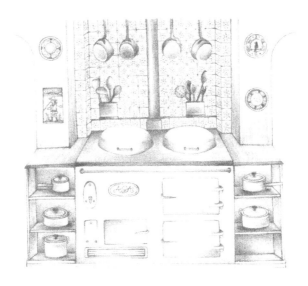

come. Next to the kitchen was a pantry with a larder full of food. In the early days of being here, Won Ton used to love sleeping in front of the Aga, because it was comforting to know that the pantry was so close by and the Aga gave off pleasing warmth. Eventually though, he exchanged the hard floor of the kitchen for the soft sofa in the lounge and the entertainment provided by the TV and console.

All day long Won Ton was free to do what he liked best and that happened to be spending hours munching away in front of the TV. Today he was watching his favourite wildlife programme, *Tropical Birds*. Didn't these cute, colourful creatures produce the most fascinating sounds! Won Ton thought. So high in pitch! Just beautiful, and how elegant they looked sailing up and down at great speed. The highlight of the show had just come up: Hummingbirds feeding on nectar. Like jewels, their feathers mesmerized him, but watching those birds made him feel hungry. All the food on the couch table had vanished. To get hold of more would mean having to leave his soft warm spot and

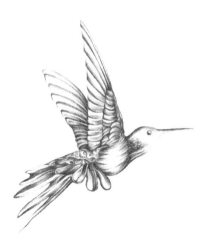

walk over to the kitchen. But his stomach was rumbling so badly! Sofa, kitchen – sofa, so good, kitchen? Kitchen. With a mighty groan he heaved himself up and waddled across to the larder where all his treasures were stored: Jellied Salmon, Lamb in Wildberry Sauce, Chicken Breast Fillets in Lobster Mousse and his ultimate delight: double cream. It took him a while to make up his mind, but in the end he went for the healthy option, the jellied salmon. He had perfected the art of opening packets with a slice of his claw. Tins were opened with a pencil inserted into the metal loop and a tug with his jaws, the tin being held down with his paws. After he finished he would take the cans or pouches to the big bins outside and hide them there so Aaron and Rebecca did not find them. He did

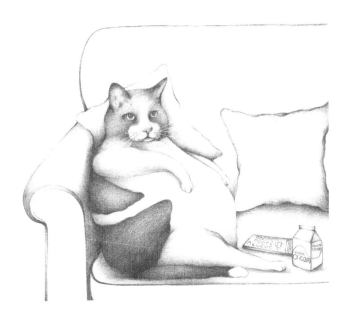

not want them to know how much he was eating in between the meals they gave him.

Those omega 3 fats are good for you! And why not? he said to himself, Some cream to wash it down with won't do any harm. Satisfied with his choice, Won Ton took his tidbits back to the living room and settled down on his beloved sofa again. All the food was gone in the flash of a wing. He considered afters. No. I've got to watch my waistline. Not that I am too fat, he reasoned. Just a little round in the middle. Won Ton was good at fooling himself. He replayed the hummingbird sequence a few times, before feeling restless. Let's see if I can just find a little something, he thought. Again Won Ton found himself inside the larder. Beaming at him from the top shelf was the can of lobster mousse. He jumped, but couldn't get anywhere near it. He tried again, this time making a run for it, but still no luck. Won Ton was out of breath. I am not giving up, he thought in despair. This stool might just do it. He climbed up onto the stool, raised his paws above his head, tottered, wobbled, almost fell off the stool and then low and behold, there he had it in his paws! But, alas, as he was trying to step down, Won Ton lost his balance and fell with a heavy thump onto his backside. The can slipped out of his paws, rolled and disappeared under the kitchen units. Oh no, what now? Despite his sore bottom Won Ton man-

aged to move himself onto his stomach to try and lo-
cate the whereabouts of the can by groping around in
the dark with his paw. Yes, he could just about feel it.
He wedged himself under the unit stretching his arms
as far forward as possible and – yes, there it was in his
paws again! Now reverse and back to my sofa pronto,
he thought! But, my goodness, he could not move
– neither forwards, nor backwards. He was jammed
in. He held his breath whilst desperately trying to
move his hind legs, only to find that he had shoved
himself further in. Now he was completely stuck. He
could hardly breathe and his legs were beginning to
feel numb. There was a horrible smell of spilled cook-
ing oil and ancient dust about. Surprised to see him, a
spider scuttled away. Won Ton grew more desperate.
Who would come to his rescue? Aaron and Rebecca
wouldn't be home until late in the evening and his
sister Hissie usually came home whenever she felt like

it. Sometimes she wouldn't be back for days. He cried for help, but to no avail. I'd better save my breath, he thought. The can, although he was still holding it so tight, was no use to him at all now. Won Ton was petrified that he might suffocate any second.

After what felt like hours, he heard a noise. The cat flap!

'Hissie! Help, Hissie, I am in the kitchen!'

There was no answer.

'Hissie, I am stuck, please help!'

Still no reply. Won Ton started to panic. I hope it's not that gate-crashing stray I gave a telling off the other day, he thought. Someone was approaching on velvety paws. Won Ton's heart was pounding and he expected the worst.

'Hi, Fatso, you've got yourself into a bit of a mess here, haven't you?' Hissie sneered.

Won Ton was so relieved, he almost cried.

'You know, your bum looks like an oversized sofa in long johns!'

'Thanks for that assessment, Sis, but could you please help me before I die from cardiac arrest or worse!'

Hissie, being as thin as a stick, slipped effortlessly under the unit to investigate the cause of her brother's mishap.

'Won Ton, is this the reason you are trapped under here?' she said, pointing to the can. That should teach you a lesson. You only think about food, nothing else. I will help you though, under one condition.

'And that condition would be?' gasped Won Ton.

'That you promise to lose weight. Am I not a good example of how to look?' Hissie lifted her chin and arched her back.

'Okay, okay, I will do whatever you want me to do, but please get me out of here,' Won Ton pleaded.

Hissie took pity at last and started to pull at his legs, but he did not budge. After tugging with all her might she managed to shift him a little. Won Ton cried out in pain.

'Won Ton, hold in your tummy and don't breathe!' Hissie said.

Feeling faint from the lack of space and oxygen, he did as he was told.

Hissie took one more deep breath, pulled again with all the strength she could muster and with a painful squelch, Won Ton was free! He was so out of breath, that he did not even have the strength to say anything in gratitude. He kept collapsing whenever he tried to get up, his legs were sore and still quite numb and his side had been scraped by the counter's edges.

Having recovered at last, though still collapsed on the floor, Won Ton was wondering whether he could ask Hissie to pull out the can that he had been forced

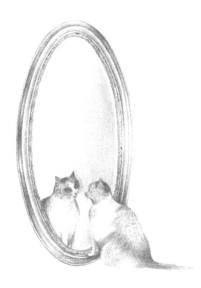

to let go of in the end.

But then he remembered his promise to her. Did he really say he would go on a diet? Hissie was sitting next to him grooming herself. She looked at her brother and shook her pretty head.

'Honestly Bro, find a mirror and then you will know what I mean.'

Won Ton dragged himself in front of the big mirror in the hall. His face was covered in cobwebs, his hindquarters appeared to have doubled in size

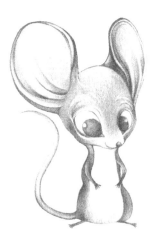

and his head looked tiny in comparison. He did not look like a cat in his teens, frankly, he felt, and looked, middle-aged. But he was too exhausted to even clean himself up.

He limped to the sofa and dragged himself up onto the soft cushions. Doesn't that feel good! he thought to himself. True, he deserved a bit of relaxation after this ordeal! How about playing a game of *Catch the Mouse*?

Whenever he played his electronic game, *Catch the Mouse*, he always tried to top his highest score.

You start off with a tiny mouse, which is impossibly small and fast and when you catch it you move on to a medium sized one who is very clever at setting up traps against the pursuer. Then at the last level, you are confronted with a giant, highly intelligent mouse, presenting you with all sorts of difficult obstacles.

'Hey Bro, you could've at least said thank you! There you go again, on your bum, playing that useless game. Well, I am off to catch real mice now,' Hissie said

She tossed her head as she headed for the front door. By the way, we have new neighbours,' she said as she headed for the old stone pillars outside the door. I believe they are from LA. I will check them

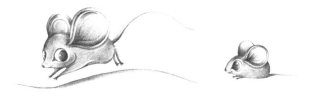

out. And don't forget your promise!' Hissie shouted
as she made her way up the slate path to the wrought
iron gate, her pert posterior swaying elegantly as she
walked.

Won Ton, totally absorbed in his game, was quite
unaware of Hissie leaving the room, he muttered
something like 'Yeah.' Suddenly he heard a strange
noise: *Brrr, brrr, rumble.*

Where did that come from? Again, *rumble, brrr,*

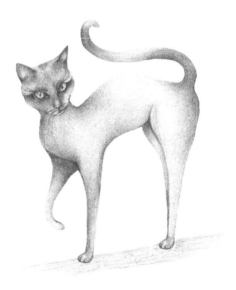

brrr. Ah, of course. It was his stomach! After such a major trauma he was starving, naturally! Won Ton got up, went to the larder and picked up as much he could carry. Back on the sofa, he greedily gobbled everything up and washed it all down with a pint of cream. Yes, that felt good!

With his tummy now fully replenished he was happy and belched contentedly. However, this heavenly state did not last for long. He remembered Hissie's words and his own promise. A promise he had just broken! A great feeling of shame shot through him, and then something unseen settled in his stomach, a sense that told him that something had to change! Yes, Won Ton was determined! I will start with my diet – tomorrow! Imagining a new, leaner him, he leaned back on the sofa and began to drift off. His game forgotten, the mouse ran in frenzied circles along a grid on the starting screen.

CHAPTER TWO

FARMYARDS, FOXES AND FRIENDSHIP

Won Ton was stirring in his sleep. He had been dreaming about a grey-skied, muddy farmyard swarming with piglets and kittens. It made Won Ton feel uneasy to see all these animals running around in a panic and his stomach turned in his sleep. To make things worse, hundreds of fox cubs appeared and dashed across the courtyard as if they had just been released from a large sack. Two chubby hands appeared out of nowhere, followed by a big, pink face. The farmer's wife, her tongue poking from the corner of her mouth in concentration!

She grabbed him by the neck and … Won Ton woke with a start. Yes, there it was again. He kept having this horrible dream that always left him feeling guilty and ashamed about whom he was. Memories of the past few years came back to him.

Won Ton, being one of seven kittens, was born in the corner of the barn next to the pigsty. It was a cold and dark place. Only when snuggling up to his brothers and sisters did he ever feel warm or loved. One day, the farmer's wife picked them up by the scruffs of their necks and took them to the rain barrel, two at a time where she proceeded to drown them with grim determination. *There are just too many of you this year, and nobody seems to want you.* Won Ton watched his siblings disappear over the lip of the barrel. Mesmerised, he stared at a rusty strip of binding hoop and wondered where they had gone and when they would be coming out again. The farmer's wife was just about to start on the second last kitten, which happened to be Hissie, when the farmer came back from the fields on his tractor.

Oi, stop it woman, are there still any left? I promised a couple to those townies in the cottage.

The image of Hissie poised in the air as the farmer's wife listened to her husband was like a photograph that Won Ton tried not to take out of his mind too often. The kittens were left skidding in the dust where the farmer's wife dumped them before she stomped away shouting, *What are they worth?*

How the words of the farmers haunted him. This was how Hissie and Won Ton stopped chasing each other's tails in a huge dusty barn with only the pigs – who ignored them, they had a *sty*, after all – and the tractor for company. As Won Ton lay on the sofa, watching the sun filter through the bay tree outside the window, the words of the farmer's wife came back to him again. *What are they worth?* What am I worth? He thought. He smothered the thought by picturing what he could have for breakfast, but then he remembered Hissie's words and felt guilty. I will do something about it, he thought to himself. Just not now.

After breakfast, and in keeping with his decision to make changes in his life, Won Ton decided to explore the big oak tree, whose branches stretched out over the back lawn and across to the fox den. He had been meaning to go up there for quite a while, but had always put it off until now. Today, spurred on by his desire to become a new, sleeker version of himself, he felt adventurous and daring, even a little reckless.

So there he was, at the bottom of this magnificent giant. He took a deep breath that extended his girth even more and began to climb the trunk. It was very hard work. Being a bit round in his midriff didn't exactly help; his tummy seemed to act as a brake on the bark of the tree. After reaching the first branch it seemed to get easier and Won Ton went higher and higher until, without thinking about it, he was almost at the top.

Feeling elated by his achievement, he sat on a forked branch and looked down for the first time. Oh dear, it was such a long way down, he could hardly make out the daisies! Won Ton suddenly felt very light headed. He was petrified that he was going to lose his balance and fall to his certain death.

What to do?

One: Sit there with his eyes tightly shut and call for help? Would somebody hear him?

Two: Sit there and wait until Hissie, Aaron or Rebecca would come looking for him? That could take ages!

Three: Positive thinking! Try to enjoy the vista of the heath and parkland and then just make your way down like a cool cat – wishful thinking.

Won Ton grew more and more desperate. Just as he thought things could not get much worse he saw the fox cubs emerge from the den – one, two, three, four of them. Won Ton's heart started to race, he had a flashback to the farm and his claws gripped the bark in terror. Now, here comes trouble! Each night the little foxes kept the whole neighbourhood awake, screeching and causing havoc and destruction; running around the back gardens, tearing open bins and playing with the contents! They started running around the tree trunk trying to catch each other's tails, whilst Won Ton, so they would not discover him, tried to make himself look small – but no such luck. They might have looked cute, they even reminded Won Ton of himself at the same age, but they were not cats. Won Ton told himself not to soften. The one with the bushiest tail and big bright eyes looked up and saw him cowering.

'Look who we've got here, guys!' he sniggered. 'It's that fatso from the mansion. Looks like he hasn't got the guts to come back down. What a loser!'

The other cubs screeched with glee. Then all three raised their tails and lifted their legs in unison against the trunk. An acrid smell wafted up to Won Ton and

he was beginning to feel sick with disgust and shame.
The fox known as Bushy Tail, whispered something
to his siblings. The three foxes then started to dance
around the oak tree chanting:

"Fat Cat is stuck, not in the mud, but in a tree.
How stupid can you be?"

On and on they went, singing their cruel rhyme.
Ashamed, Won Ton wanted to cover his ears, but he
was scared of losing his grip. A sudden booming voice
silenced them instantly.

'Now, you three troublemakers! Did I not tell you
to stay in the den until your mother and I were back!'

The fox cubs stood still and their tails
drooped.

'Off you go at once, I'll deal with you later!'

Their tails hanging and their faces staring at the
ground, one by one they turned round and followed
their mother, who stood at the entrance to the den,

her eyes stern as she looked at them over her shoulder.

'Sorry about this, old chap!' yelled father fox up to Won Ton. 'This lot are really out of control at the moment. I will go and get some help from the mansion, as I'm afraid I cannot climb trees. Help will be there in no time, and that is a promise from Methuselah, your friendly fox and neighbour!'

Won Ton wanted to thank him, but he had a big lump in his throat, so only a hoarse whisper escaped

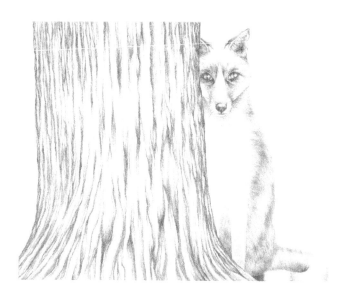

his mouth. As he crouched, wind shivered at his whiskers, making him sink his claws ever deeper into the bark of his branch. Methuselah ran to the back door and opened and closed the cat flap as noisily as he could until he heard footsteps on the stairs. As soon as Aaron appeared at the door, Met ran back towards the tree, gave Won Ton his thumbs up and seemingly vanished into thin air. Aaron, who had been washing up, looked out the window and spotted something black and white at the top of the oak tree and heard a faint call for help.

'Won Ton!' Aaron shouted as he grabbed the big ladder from the side of the house and carried it to the tree, only to realise that it would be far too short. Won Ton thought he was doomed. I'll never get down from here again!

'Won Ton, hold on!' Aaron called up to him. 'I am going to call the fire brigade, okay? Don't let go!'

A few minutes later Won Ton could hear the sound of a siren coming closer. Four firemen stormed into the garden carrying all sorts of equipment and an extendable ladder. One of them, a stocky guy with a kind sort of face shouted up to him in a broad London accent.

'Hi mate, name's Gary! Hold on alright, be right with you!' The ladder was extended and Gary quickly climbed to the top. Won Ton saw him coming closer and closer until he was right in front of him. 'I'll put you in the harness now mate. You're alright.'

Won Ton was so overwhelmed that he burst into tears. Gary gently lifted him off the branch and put him in the harness close to his chest.

'There you go mate, we'll be down in no time!'

Won Ton, all safe and sound on Gary's chest now, was not so scared of the height anymore.

When he was finally back on the ground, Won Ton

could not stop hugging and thanking him. He twirled himself round and round Gary's legs, purring. The rest of the firemen gave him a big cheer. As quickly as they had come they rushed out with all their gear back to the waiting engine and left with a street audience of neighbours to cheer them on their way.

Aaron was hugely relieved that Won Ton was uninjured and lifted him gently into his arms.

'You are getting heavy aren't you? But we do love you,' Aaron snuggled up to Won Ton and the world seemed right again.

Aaron could not wait to tell Rebecca about the rescue operation. As they moved back into the house, Won Ton thought of that magnificent fox again. Without him I probably would have starved to death up there, he thought.

He felt faint with exhaustion and … hunger!

After his first encounter with Methuselah, Won Ton

went into the back garden, week in week out, hoping to meet him again. Often he would sit for hours under the dense growth of ivy close to the den, waiting.

Finally, his patience was rewarded. It was already getting dark and the crescent of the moon had made an appearance in the sky when Won Ton saw Methuselah creep through the fence. Won Ton, overjoyed to see him, shot out of the ivy to greet him.

'Methuselah, I'm not sure whether you remember me. I am the cat that got stuck in the tree, how stupid can you be!' – he left out the rest.

'Of course I remember you. How are you? I can see you have turned into a fully-grown tom since we last met.

'Well, it actually dawned on me, that I never had a chance to thank you properly. That's why I waited for you to let you know how very grateful I am and that I will never forget what you have done for me. Thank you, thank you, thank you!'

'That's quite alright, any time! But listen, I've got to go. Urgent business to attend to. Good to see you again, Big Tom Tiger.' Methuselah hurried towards his den.

Won Ton felt his happiness draining away like the light from the sky as he stood and watched him go. He had waited so long for this encounter! But as Methuselah was just about to disappear into his den he turned around again. There was something touching about this earnest and sincere chap, with a slightly forlorn air about him, he thought. He turned round.

'Look, whenever you want to speak to me and need help, come here and whistle three times.'

Feeling very honoured, Won Ton blushed up to his whiskers that Methuselah was offering his guidance and friendship to him.

'That means the world to me, Met, if I may call you

that. And I will practice whistling, not my strongest point!'

Met waved his paw and vanished down into the den.

Of course he would only consult him if there were a real crisis, as Met was a busy fox with a whole family and community on his hands! With a spring in his step, Won Ton went back to his house.

CHAPTER THREE

THE BEST DIET STARTS

TOMORROW

Memories of the time before his and Hissie's lucky escape from the farmyard kept coming back to haunt Won Ton, leaving him with feelings of emptiness and guilt. Why had he survived when his brothers and sisters had not? What had happened to his mother? And why was it all coming back with such force now? He felt abandoned by his mother even though he knew she was as much a victim of the farmers as he and Hissie were. The feeling of emptiness that arose when these thoughts drifted into his mind would drive him to eating, sometimes until he felt like he would explode, but he would still feel empty, even though his tummy was almost bursting. When he thought about his childhood mistreatment the only solace seemed to be switching on the TV and trying to switch off his feelings – with something from the fridge. Curling himself around his owner's legs usually did the trick, especially if there was a can to be opened – he only performed his pouch and can tricks when his owners were out as he did not want them to know about his secret eating.

He was quite good at whistling now and Met kept to his promise to respond when he was home and they had become good friends. Won Ton had sought Met's advice a few times when his childhood burden almost seemed to crush his soul and his friend's advice had become a source of nourishment to him. Every time he left the den, he did so in a better state of mind. As Met often said, *it's good to talk*. Met tried to keep Won Ton's spirits up by telling him that it was understandable that he felt as he did and that he was a survivor. He told him that life was a gift that he should cherish, and that he owed it to Hissie and his siblings to make something of his life.

But despite all the meetings and the well-meant advice Won Ton still felt empty much of the time. He had not yet come to realise that he was the one who could take charge and bring change to his life.

Won Ton waddled to the larder again and stuffed himself, his promise to Hissie momentarily forgotten, but more and more he was becoming aware that he was not achieving the expected satisfaction. Trying to distract himself he decided to go out into the garden. He squeezed through the cat flap and almost got stuck!

As he approached his favourite camellia shrub he noticed voices in the rose garden. It was Hissie, deep in conversation with another cat, or rather what was left of it. More like a furry skeleton!

'Oh, Barbie, you must tell me all about this Californian diet! I need to shed a few pounds here and there.' Hissie must be joking; she doesn't need to lose any weight! At her whiskers perhaps, Won Ton thought.

In a broad American accent this grotesque creature called Barbie said:

'Darling, it is the easiest thing in the world. Keep telling yourself that you are free from food. I don't need food and food doesn't need me! Keep repeating this as soon as you are tempted! Who needs to eat anyway, only weaklings and losers? If you get really, really hungry, eat as much as you can, as quickly as you can. After that … paw down the throat and problem solved!'

'That sounds pretty straightforward to me,' Hissie replied. But how do you stop yourself from catching mice? It's in our genetic makeup!'

'Oh, it's all a matter of discipline, dear,' Barbie said. 'You play with them, and when they are dead, you just lick their blood. That keeps the iron deficiency, and the calories under control, Sweetie.'

Hissie seemed a bit alarmed at hearing about iron

deficiency for the first time, and her green eyes widened, but then she looked jealously at Barbie's Figure. She wanted to look like her, elegant, glamorous and with legs to die for!

Won Ton almost felt sick after hearing what he did. How ghastly, to make yourself sick after eating! What is the point of catching mice and then make do with licking their blood! That's like having Sunday roast without the roast! What a miserable existence!

Hissie had all she could ever wish for! A beautiful shiny black coat, eyes like emeralds and a perfect body, Won Ton thought. He had to save his sister and make her not listen to this skinny minx with her grey coat and her bulging eyes.

Won Ton emerged from the shrubbery and cried out: 'Hissie, can you come here for a mo?' Both cats were startled and looked at him. Barbie started to giggle, the giggle becoming more and more hysterical.

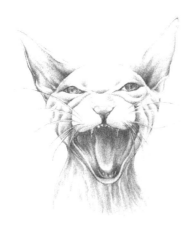

Between gasps, she cried, 'Oh my goodness, you really haven't promised too much. Your brother looks like a Big Mac on stumps!' As Barbie was on the point of collapse, Won Ton noticed that half of her teeth were missing, which made her look ghoulish.

He pretended to ignore her and just addressed Hissie.

'Listen, Hissie, come home with me now. Come on, sis', you don't want this.'

Hissie felt terribly embarrassed about her obese brother. 'I come home whenever it pleases me and this is none of your business!' she hissed. 'Just look at you, you blob.'

Barbie was still in a fit of hysterics, rolling on the lawn and exposing her rotten teeth. Won Ton went right up to her face, giving her his widest smile and showing his perfect, white cogs.

'Nice meeting you too. I am Hissie's twin, by the way, and if anybody tries to harm her I can get quite nasty!'

'Twin?' Barbie stopped laughing immediately, turned the other way and sulked.

'How dare you insult my friend like this,' Hissie snarled.

Now Won Ton was offended. He meant well after all and for once was standing up for his sister. And look what he got in return!

'Honestly, Hissie, can't say I haven't tried, but if you want to starve yourself to death, go on then, hope you enjoy yourself!' Won Ton turned around with as much dignity as he could muster and went back to the house, feeling lonely and misunderstood.

As he padded to his favourite spot on the sofa, the realisation that things had to change solidified in his mind. He would show Hissie that he could do it! He recalled an advert he had seen on TV the other day. This guy was praising a new product that guaranteed weight loss for cats. It was called *Tom Trim*.

There was no other way out Won Ton decided. He considered that he was meant to see that advert. He would have to go and find this stuff somewhere. Yes, tomorrow he would head off into a new life! He ran back up the garden and up the white steps leading to the cat flap with a spring in his admittedly wobbly paw steps.

CHAPTER FOUR

NEW ARRIVALS AND NEW

BEGINNINGS

After his upsetting encounter with Hissie and Barbie, Won Ton faced a restless night. He tossed and turned before he fell into a troubled sleep. He dreamed about climbing a ladder. Up and up he went towards the sky.

When he was about to reach the clouds, the rungs cracked under his weight, he lost his grip, and fell down in slow motion. Just as he was about to hit the ground he heard a high-pitched bark. Won Ton woke up in a cold sweat, his heart beating fast. He immediately sensed that something was not quite right. There were unfamiliar noises in the kitchen. Apart from Rebecca and Aaron's voices he could hear some yapping and whining.

With stiff limbs and a faint headache, Won Ton got up to find out what was going on. The kitchen door was ajar and he glimpsed Rebecca cooing over a little black creature with bats ears in her arms. Worse, Aar-

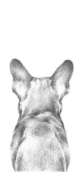

on was feeding massive chunks of meat to a big white furry creature. Was it a wolf? Surely, he must still be in a bad dream!

Tentatively he pushed open the door. As he did so, Rebecca shouted, 'Hold on to her collar, Aaron!'

But the big, white wolf had already spotted him and, with bared teeth, darted towards Won Ton. As Won Ton turned, he found himself being chased out of the back door and into the garden, closely pursued by this barking monster. The indignity!

He was running for his life! His only hope was

Methuselah's den. Won Ton darted towards the dense ivy and disappeared down into the tunnel. There he cowered, trying not to make any noise, which was well nigh impossible due to the heaving of his breath. He could hear the ghastly beast sniffing and scratching! Won Ton's heart beat fast and furiously. Any minute now his number was up, he thought. There was a distant rumble of thunder. The wolf stopped as if he had been struck by something and bolted back to the house, howling, tail between its legs.

Phew, what a relief it's gone! But what is happening? Won Ton thought. Why are Rebecca and Aaron turning up with bat-eared dogs and wolves? Is this some kind of a joke? Won Ton was really annoyed! I

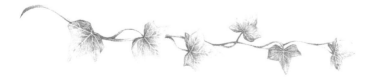

mean, here I am, embarking on a new life to acquire a dream body and the perfect life and now I'm being chased out of my own house by monsters!

Still, this was not going to stop him trying to get hold of this wonder food. Nothing will stop me! I will prove I can do it to myself and to Hissie! Hissie – he had to warn her about this canine invasion!

First things first though, he thought. I need to get hold of Met. He whistled three times and anxiously waited for Met's footsteps. Nothing! Let's try again. This time his whistle sounded more like a rusty old drainpipe. There was another rumble of thunder a bit closer by. He felt more and more desperate, lonely and scared. I can't even go home, please Met, where are you? After what felt like a lifetime, he could hear Met scrambling up the deep tunnel. There he was, with his wise face and what Won Ton now saw was his failing body. He was quite concerned when he noticed that his ribs were standing out even more and his coat had more bald patches then last time. But Met's eyes still had their old sparkle. Won Ton got up with a sigh of relief to meet his friend and guardian.

'Oh, Met!' he cried, relieved.

'Hello, old chap,' Met, replied. 'What is the matter? You don't quite look yourself, tell me what's up?'

Won Ton told him about Hissie and Barbie making fun of him for his size and that he was determined to go on a diet. Met, who had listened to Won Ton thoughtfully, asked if he always thought about food and why.

'It is always good to find out why we do things, old chap. Once we know the why, we can look at the why not,' Met winked at him.

Nobody had ever asked him that question before! If he had known the answer, Won Ton would proba- bly not have been sitting in a fox den. When he related the story about being chased down the garden by this ghastly wolf dog that seemed to have taken his place, Won Ton broke down in tears. Met who had grown very fond of this lovely fellow, felt really sorry for Won Ton. He gave him a hug, followed by a pat on his back.

'Nothing we can't sort out together,' he said. After a few more sobs, Won Ton blew his nose and, strangely enough, felt much better. A sense of hope was forming in his heart that made him feel almost light.

'A problem shared is a problem aired,' said Methuselah. 'And once aired, it can be dispelled – one way or another. Where there is a will there is a way.'

'Well, Met, speaking of *will* I've got a favour to ask. Could you please help me get hold of this new diet stuff? I don't have a clue where to go. It's called *Tom Trim*. I saw an ad about it the other day …'

Met scratched his head, as he pondered where the

best place to get diet food from might be. Then he re-membered. 'Yes, I think I know exactly the place you are looking for. It's called *The Jolly Chickpea* and it's not far from here. When times got really bad, I used to go through their bins, but what I found tasted like horse manure!'

'Oh, Met, what would I do without you! You are simply the best!'

'Okay, Big Tom Tiger Won Ton, let's find the Jolly Chickpea. Follow me down the tunnel!'

Won Ton jumped up in anticipation and followed Met's skinny tail, into the bright future that now seemed within his reach.

CHAPTER FIVE

THE WARREN

'Stay close, it is a maze down here,' Met disappeared down a dark, narrow underground passage and Won Ton followed suit.

It was pretty airless and narrow in the earthen passages of the warren and the deeper they went the more suffocated he felt. Won Ton found himself thinking of the cosy sofa back home, envisioning the tasty treats in the pantry, but then he thought of the dogs, and, despite the stench, he took a deep breath and pressed on, following Met's tail with his glistening eyes. The passage he was in had lots of turnings off to the left and right and soon Won Ton totally lost his sense of direction. After what seemed a very long time the passage opened up and they seemed to have reached the heart of the warren.

'Welcome to my humble home, or what's left of it,' Methuselah said.

Won Ton sank down onto the ground that was

littered with bones and feathers.

There was a funny, sweet smell in the chamber and a definite lack of oxygen. Met went scavenging through a heap of bones and torn up rubbish and pulled out a half eaten drumstick which he held right under Won Ton's nose. He was so ravenous he nearly took it, despite it being off. But he thought better of it.

'No, thank you, Met. You need it more than I do, besides, remember why we are on this mission?'

'Just wanted to find out if you meant business, my friend!' Met wolfed down the drumstick in one big gulp, before wiping his whiskers and giving Won Ton

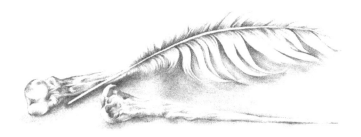

a big wink.

Won Ton was pretty exhausted and dreaded the second part of their journey through this dark, airless maze, but after a few minutes rest, Met made him get up again. Up, down, left, down and right they went. Won Ton was on the brink of turning round when Met called out, 'This is the last bit. It's quite steep, so hold on to my tail!'

Met almost fell backwards as Won Ton clung to his tail. However, slowly but surely Met lifted Won Ton up the steep tunnel and, with his last strength pulled him out of the warren. Both of them collapsed onto the ground struggling for air as torrential rain belted onto them. To Won Ton, it felt like an embrace.

After getting his bearings again, Won Ton found himself in a big yard. It was full of overflowing wheel-ie bins, old furniture and scrap metal. Won Ton was about to suggest that they seek some shelter under one of the wheelie bins when a bolt of lightening, followed by a crash of thunder made him dart underneath the biggest one. He called on Met to follow suit. He felt much safer now and peeked out to see what had taken his friend so long.

What he saw made the blood freeze in his veins. A gigantic fox had appeared and was blocking Met's way. His teeth were bared and his yellow eyes were full of malice as he pawed the ground in front of Methuselah.

'Ah, it's you, Brutus. Thought I recognized that stink from somewhere!' Met said mildly.

'What are you doing in *my* territory, you old fool? Thought you were a goner, rotting away in a dump! Look at you, what a pathetic sight!' Brutus said.

Methuselah had seen this coming for some time. Brutus had been meaning to challenge his leadership for a while, but the timing could not have been worse.

'Well, well, Brutus, *your* territory! It is a well-known fact that I am in charge of these realms. Besides you have to play by the rules if you want to challenge me!'

'Rules! Brutus was spitting out the word! You play by *my* rules!'

Won Ton watched in horror as the two foxes started to circle around each other. He wanted to jump out of his hiding place and somehow prevent what he knew was going to happen, but he was paralysed with fear.

The storm had eased up a bit, but the atmosphere was highly charged. Methuselah realized that Brutus was much younger and stronger than himself. He had to find his weak spot.

'Come on then, Brutus, what are you waiting for. Getting cold feet? You know, the fox population is quite aware of the fact, that you are not exactly the brightest star of our community. Quite the laughing stock!'

With a distorted expression Brutus charged towards Met.

'Ha, I got him. Vanity,' Met thought, but instantly he was thrown onto his back. Brutus pinned him down to the ground whilst Met tried desperately to kick him in the groin, but without success.

Brutus sank his teeth into Met's throat, severing an artery. Blood gushed out onto the dusty ground, but he felt no pain. For a split second Brutus lost his grip and Met went straight for his nose. Brutus yelped in pain. I have to get on top of him, Met thought, but Brutus held him down in an iron grip, going for the wound in his throat again. Met thought of his family and what a blessed life he had lived. With unexpected strength he freed his upper body and ripped off Brutus' ear. Brutus was caught by surprise and with a glazed expression, looked at his severed ear; not realizing it actually belonged to him. Met took advantage of his puzzlement and with his last might pushed him off and jumped onto his back in a flash, his old bones still remembered the canniest battle moves. Brutus tried to shake him off, but, with an experienced twist, Met turned his head anti-clockwise. A horrible cracking sound filled the back yard. Brutus's body rose up in an arch, his head lolling from side to side; he crashed down onto the ground and into a puddle, his eyes already empty. Brutus was gone. Won Ton was trembling from top to bottom. For a moment, he could not move, and the dark night of his soul seemed to have tightened its grip on him. Slowly at first, Won Ton crawled out from under the bin, but then hurried to his friend's side, tears streaming down his face. Smiling weakly, Met was standing next to the dead Brutus. As Won Ton reached him, his hind legs gave way and he fell into Won Ton's arms. The rain had stopped and there was just a distant rumble of thunder. Won Ton put Met gently to the ground, stroking his head.

'Met, let me get you something to make you more comfortable.' Won Ton was distraught and frantically tried to find something suitable in the filthy yard.

In the far corner he spotted a damp discarded curtain, which he carefully slipped under Met's body.

'There you go, that will make you feel better. Met, you were amazing. You are still the king of all the foxes in North London and beyond!'

'Won Ton, you have to complete your journey by yourself,' Met said, lifting his head slightly. 'You will be fine, Met! We'll just wait until you have recovered and the bleeding has stopped!' Won Ton, pleaded.

As he looked at the gaping wound in his friend's throat, Won Ton realised, that Met was fatally injured. This must not happen, no! Without him he would not go anywhere, he would rather die with him! In a faint whisper Met said, Listen to me, Tame Tiger Won Ton, follow your path and don't give up. You have come a long way and now you must complete your journey. I will watch over you.'

Met took one more rattling breath, then his body relaxed and a peaceful expression spread over his wise face.

Won Ton threw himself on top of Met's body; big bitter tears were streaming down his face. It's all my fault! Why did I not come to his rescue? I am such a coward, such a disgrace! Won Ton was still lying on top of his friend's body, when he heard a scuttling noise coming nearer and nearer. Looking up he saw a massive rat sniffing the air, followed by a few smaller ones. This was too much for him! Angrily he wiped away his tears and charged towards them. 'Shoo, you vile creatures. Leave us alone, get away from here before I slaughter you one by one!'

The rats rapidly scurried back into the shadows.

Won Ton had to do something about his friend's body. He looked around. I have to put him somewhere safe, he thought. On a heap of scrap metal he found a broken shovel and, working steadily, Won Ton dug a shallow grave. Exhausted, he draped the curtain around Met's body and lowered him into the ground. He mounted the soil on top and made a cross out of two sticks, he marked the grave with his claws: R.I.P. Methuselah. Strangely enough, this made Won Ton feel better. He was not a coward after all. He had defended him, found the strength to bury him and now he would follow his path. Yes, he would carry on. Won Ton walked out of the yard towards a little alley, just as the sun was making an appearance through the clouds.

CHAPTER SIX

MARBLE, LIGHTS, CRYSTAL, AND STONE

Barbie had moved to London only four weeks ago and was quite pleased to have found such a perfect target in her neighbourhood. She relished telling that gullible thing Hissie all the tricks of her trade as they strutted along the pavement! She thought about her journey from the USA. What a horrible flight it had been! The airhostess had insisted on Barbie traveling in that silly basket. Me, prize winning Barbie! That certainly wasn't the kind of treatment she was used to. After all, she had won nearly all the beauty contests up and down the West Coast! Here in London she was facing an uncertain future, but she kept up the boasting and never lost an opportunity to compare London unfavourably to LA, and all this despite the fact that her health was deteriorating, as were her teeth.

The thunderstorm was coming closer and Barbie suggested that she and Hissie go to her house to avoid the rain. Hissie felt flattered to be invited home by this

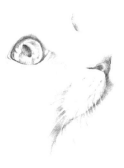

super cool new friend. As the two of them walked on Hissie noticed a big tomcat sitting under the porch of a red-brick mansion block.

He was very handsome cat with a lean, but strong body and bright blue eyes. As they walked past him, he pulled a face whilst looking at Barbie, but gave Hissie a keen smile and a wink. She pretended not to have noticed him and walked on self-consciously, with strangely stiff legs. The sirens of a police car and an ambulance distracted Barbie, who was not quite used to London life yet. Her eyes bulged and Hissie looked concerned.

Just before they turned into Barbie's street, they had to dodge three miniature poodles and their slightly flustered owner on the way to the new dog parlour.

'Honestly, some people have no respect,' Barbie said irately. The poodles yapped at them and Barbie hissed.

'How dare you!' the lady poodle owner said, her large sunglasses bearing down on them.

Barbie glared at her and the two giggled

Hissie could not believe her eyes when they arrived at Barbie's place. Behind unobtrusive front doors was a massive mansion. Walking through the front door she was almost blinded. There were mirrors everywhere. The floor was made of shiny black marble and the furniture of glass and chrome. Huge chandeliers

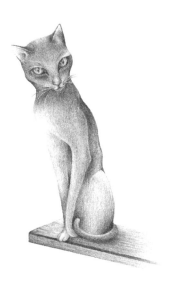

shone from the ceiling. Barbie was admiring herself in front of a gigantic mirror. When Hissie noticed her own reflection next to her, she got a nasty shock. Oh, my goodness, I look so fat next to her! From now on, I won't touch a single crumb until I look exactly like her, she thought.

'Darling, I've got a question,' Barbie said. 'Back in California, we have pet dentists. You see, I've lost quite a few of my teeth now,' Barbie tilted her head, 'because, well you know why, for a good cause, and was wondering whether you have them in this country too?'

Hissie was puzzled. Is this the price one had to pay for starving and being sick following food? But she brushed the thought aside and replied: 'I don't know, but I'll keep my eyes and ears open. By the way, Barbie, I am absolutely starving. How do you cope with this empty stomach and being hungry all the time?'

'Easy-peasy, dear. I'll show you all the tricks. The important thing is to distract yourself! Let's paint our claws.' Barbie jumped up, but, feeling slightly light-headed, she nearly fell over.

'Are you alright?' Hissie asked anxiously.

'I am fine, dear, it's my blood pressure playing up a bit!'

As Barbie was breathing deeply in and out Hissie could not help but notice a funny smell of decay. On they went down a long corridor and through into a vast bathroom. Again there were mirrors from top to bottom and shiny tiles everywhere. Barbie opened a cabinet that was filled with hundreds of bottles of nail varnish of every colour imaginable.

'Just choose a colour, Sweetie,' Barbie said. 'I personally feel like blue today, as it matches the colour of my eyes.'

Hissie went for green to match hers. They left the bathroom and disappeared into another door at end of the corridor. Hissie gasped in amazement. Never ever had she seen such a vast space. There were three windows reaching from floor to ceiling, a four-poster bed, a treadmill and also a medical scale.

At home I have to share a saggy sofa with my obese brother and Barbie has all of this to herself, Hissie thought jealously. Thoughts such as these had become more frequent since she had been hanging out with Barbie.

The walls were covered with photos of Barbie holding up her various trophies. Barbie opened one of the built in cupboard doors and Hissie almost fainted. Collars of every style were dangling from golden hooks.

There were stripy ones, dotted ones, some with hearts and fur and others that sparkled with what looked like real diamonds. Barbie reached for the most expensive looking collar and put it on. Hissie felt very ordinary with her worn out collar and the round disc displaying her name and phone number.

They both settled onto on the big bed that was covered with a pink, fluffy throw and soft toy cats. Barbie unscrewed the bottle of varnish and started to expertly paint her claws.

Hissie, doing this for the first time, and feeling rather weak, as she always seemed to be feeling these days, struggled to open hers. Only after several attempts and twisting hard did she succeed and, with a shaky paw, she started to paint her claw. But, alas, half of it went onto her coat.

Barbie gave her a gleeful smile, which really upset Hissie. Is this how a friend behaves? she asked herself. The second claw looked much better, but when she tried to put the brush back into the bottle, it toppled over and the green nail varnish oozed out all over the pink throw. Hissie, in a desperate attempt to mop it all up, took one of the fluffy toy cats to hand and started to rub violently.

'You stupid thing!' Barbie yelled. 'What have you done!'

Hissie rubbed harder and harder, but the stain got bigger and bigger. 'Out of my bed, you brainless beast!' she shouted and then slapped Hissie right in her face.

Hissie surprised herself by hitting back, leaving a

big scratch on Barbie's nose. For a moment Barbie was stunned, so Hissie took the opportunity to get away fast. She darted out of the vast, cold room and sped down the endless corridor, her claws skidding on the marble surfaces. Barbie pursued her, all the while screeching all sorts of insults at her. At last Hissie got to the front door, but it wouldn't open. Barbie was coming closer and closer.

In her wild panic Hissie noticed the key in the door lock. She turned it and, thankfully, the door gave way. She slammed it shut behind her and, with a big sigh of relief, began to run along the wet pavement towards home.

CHAPTER SEVEN

THE JOLLY CHICKPEA

In the meantime Won Ton was walking down a busy road. He was wriggling in and out between the many shoppers but no one seemed to notice him beneath the Marks and Spencer's bags. People were too drawn in by the many attractive things displayed in the shop windows. The air smelled heavenly of pizza, cake and coffee. He was just passing a big window when he stopped dead. Cream cakes were stacked up on top of each other; there were hundreds of profiteroles, gateaux, fruit tartlets and right in the middle: a Pavlova oozing with cream! Longingly, Won Ton pressed his face against the window. After all he had been through, he deserved a little treat! Sorry, Met! His only thought was how to get into this heavenly place. The shop was almost empty. He had to wait until more customers were inside. Then he would slip in and just grab a cream cake or two. Won Ton was absolutely ravenous. He waited and waited. He sent up a silent prayer. Please, send me some people through that door! Just at that very moment, a group of school children was approaching the bakery. After a short discussion to do with who had enough money on them and who didn't and a squabble over borrowing, they entered. Won Ton was dumbfounded that Met had seemingly granted him his wish so quickly. He cast his eyes up to the sky. Thank you; I promise this is the very last time! Won Ton took another peep through the window, making sure the ladies behind the counter were busy serving the kids.

His moment had come. He sneaked through the door, jumped onto the display window and loaded as many cream cakes as he could carry into his paws. Nobody had noticed him. But, when he was about to step down, he lost his balance.

He knocked over the Pavlova and, with a splash, berries, meringues and cream cakes were sent in all directions! One of the ladies who had a face like a bulldog, and seemed about to act like one too gaped at him, absolutely horrified.

Turning scarlet she shouted, 'Oi, you! What are you doing in my shop, you monster of a cat?' she darted towards him, wielding a broom and yelling, 'Thief, thief! Catch the thief!'

Won Ton bolted out of the bakery, dropping half of his cream cakes in the process and then darted like lightning through the shoppers into the next side road. Behind a little kiosk he collapsed, gasping for breath.

When he got his breath back, Won Ton gobbled down what was left of the cream cakes. It was heavenly! Never ever in his life had anything tasted so good! Now he could think straight again and carry on searching for the Jolly Chickpea.

Back on the main road Won Ton could still hear the raised voice of the bulldog lady. Having walked for a mile or so he arrived at a T-junction and on the other side he saw an illuminated sign. *The Jolly Chickpea.*

Won Ton waited at the zebra crossing and walked over when everyone else was crossing. He had made it!

Looking through the shop window Won Ton saw all sorts of dreary looking things. Pillboxes of all sizes, vitamin supplements, some liquid that looked vile in plastic bottles, as well as orthopaedic slippers that were all scattered haphazardly over the display area. Well, I very much preferred the look of the bakery, he thought. Won Ton took a deep breath and entered. Strange and unknown smells lingered in the air. It was

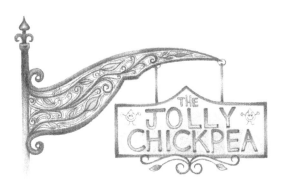

utter chaos.

Inside, the shelves were stacked so tightly with vitamins, supplements and medicine bottles, that it was probably well nigh impossible to find anything. Half open boxes littered the floor, blocking the way to the counter. It did not help either that it was quite dark inside. Only one feeble bulb dangled from the ceiling.

In order to get to the counter at the back, Won Ton had to step over quite a few baskets containing shrivelled up fruit and vegetables as well as boxes of various shampoos on special offer. Suddenly a shadow appeared behind an enormous, ancient till. A spindly, middle-aged man appeared, cleaning his glasses with the hem of a once white coat. Only after he had put the glasses back on his rather long nose, did he realize that he had a customer with a difference. Never in his life had he seen such a fat cat – not that cats were his usual clients anyway! But – the customer is always right!

He put on his winning business smile and asked, 'How can I help?'

Won Ton did not expect such a deep voice from this skinny man and felt quite awkward. 'Good day, 'erm, I was wondering whether you might have heard about this new diet food everyone is talking about. It's called, 'erm, Tom Trim?'

'Oh yes, you have come to the right place. It's just the sort of thing for our feline friends. I only got it in a few days ago and you happen to be the first to ask for it. I'll have to fetch it from the back, though. As you can see, I'm rather short of space.' He disappeared through a little door.

Won Ton heard some shuffling and creaking noises and soon enough the little man was back, carrying a big plastic bag.

'This is the best product of its kind,' he said engagingly. 'You can eat as much as you like and as often as you like … but only this, nothing else! It is the price you pay to get back on the straight and narrow, after that, you will most likely make the right decisions for yourself,' he continued in his deep, melodious voice. 'I also strongly recommend an exercise regime as diets alone leave you flabby. This one actually worked for me as well, when I was going through a round stage in my life. Nowadays, I know what to eat and how to eat. This is the individual question that must be answered by each of us.'

Won Ton could not visualize the jolly chickpea man ever having had any weight issues, but never mind that. He looked at the copy of the instructions that the man handed him as he read them out:

"'Week one, five Minutes running, then three minutes walking followed by ten press ups. Three times daily. Week two, ten minutes running, five minutes walking and twenty press-ups three times daily. Week three, fifteen Minutes running, eight minutes walking followed by three press ups three times daily. Thereafter as much running and walking and floor exercise or Callanetics or any sport you fancy up to two hours daily, three to times a week.'" He looked up. 'Any Questions?'

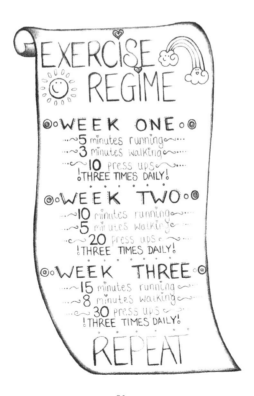

Won Ton nodded automatically, as he had lost track of what the man just told him. 'Sounds like an awful lot of exercise!' he said looking at the big plastic bag with a sense of foreboding. Brown pellets showed through a grey background of plastic.

'Anything else I can help you with?'

Won Ton just shook his head, because his throat felt slightly constricted. So the shopkeeper turned to his massive till and typed in a figure. It went ping and showed £85.00! Oh, no! Won Ton had forgotten about a tiny detail. Money! What now? He had to think of something fast, really fast; otherwise this whole venture was for nothing. With a jolt to his tummy he thought about Met, wishing he were by his side now. He would come up with a cunning plan! And then the thought came to him. I just have to tell the truth. That is what Met would have done.

With a slightly quivering voice he said, 'Dear Mr

Chickpea, I am a poor cat and on my journey to you a dear friend passed away. I will do anything to pay my debts. But will you please let me have the bag and help me become a healthy member of the feline species. I will promise to come and help you in the shop, scrub the floor or do whatever needs doing?'

Mr Chickpea – his real name was actually Jonathan – looked sternly at this big cat chap! There was such earnestness about him; he couldn't help being touched by it.

'Well, you should have thought about the money before coming here,' he said dryly. 'But I can see your good intentions and being the first customer to buy this product I will declare you my guinea pig!'

Guinea pig! Won Ton did not fancy being compared to a creature he would only ever consider as a starter or a snack!

'Come back in three months time and show me

that you have been successful. Then we take it from there. Deal? "

'That's a deal! I promise that I will be only half of myself in three months time. Thank you, Mr Chickpea, Thank you!'

Won Ton hurried home, his heart full of the warmth of human kindness. It wasn't until he got to the front gate that he found himself feeling bad and guilty for stealing the cakes. But I am not that cat anymore, he said to himself. Now that I have been to the Jolly Chickpea, there is no turning back for this cat! I will honour myself and others.

CHAPTER EIGHT

MY HOME IS MY CASTLE

Hissie was running down the road. Luckily the thunderstorm had just passed. But there were puddles of rainwater everywhere and she had to zigzag the pavement in order to avoid them. She hated water. I hope no one is going to see me like this, she thought, feeling quite vulnerable with her paws full of nail varnish.

She made it to the front of her house without anybody noticing her. What a relief! When she slipped through the sliding gate something white and furry jumped out at her, barking furiously. Hissie acted on instinct and pulled out her razor sharp claws – thank goodness they were not glued up. She repeatedly struck the creature on its nose and cheek, leaving deep

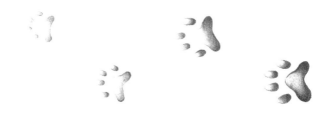

scratch marks behind. The creature – was it a dog or a wolf? – was howling now and holding his bleeding nose whilst trying to escape back into the house. Aaron had been alerted by the racket outside and quickly opened the front door. The creature ran inside, tail between legs, followed by Hissie, but with her tail right up.

'Hello, Hissie-Missie, you put somebody in her place. Well done! Sorry you had to meet like this, but we are helping out a friend of mine, who had to go into hospital. He did not know where to leave his two dogs,' Aaron said as he held the door open wide for Hissie.

And sure enough, a tiny black dog with bat-ears ran towards Hissie, and greeted her like a long lost friend. Honestly, what next? Her lethal claws came out again ready to strike, but the little dog slumped to the ground, playing dead. Hissie ignored this pathetic fur bag and marched indignantly on in the direction of the lounge.

She was very relieved that Aaron, in all the chaos, had not noticed the state she was in. How grateful she was to be back home! What a day it had been! She jumped up on top of the saggy sofa and tried to clean herself up, licking and gnawing her paws to rid herself of the varnish. It tasted awful and made her feel rather woozy. Having little success with it, her initial relief to be back home turned into anger. Red-hot anger!

How could that have happened to her! What an error of judgment to trust that horrible creature, Barbie! Being humiliated like this! And then coming home to her safe haven, and being confronted with two mad dogs!

Who makes the right decisions – I do? Who defends their territory? I do. Does anyone care about me? Nobody does. Does anyone support me? Nobody does. Am I angry and frustrated? Yes, I am! Would it be best to end it all? Yes, it would. Hissie abandoned herself to her increasingly common downward spiral.

Just as Hissie was finishing her question and answer session, Aaron popped his head around the door to say, that he was taking the dogs for a walk on the Heath and to meet Rebecca for a drink at their local pub afterwards. Hissie was quite happy to have the place to herself. That did not happen very often.

Actually, where is Won Ton? He was usually always at home. Hissie realised she missed him, but quickly snuffed the thought out and made another attempt to get the remaining nail varnish off before giving up. She was ravenous! Come to think of it, she had not eaten anything proper in days. Feeling pretty light headed she leapt off the sofa and walked over to the larder. There she helped herself to a tin of salmon, and grabbing the stem of a teaspoon, opened it with

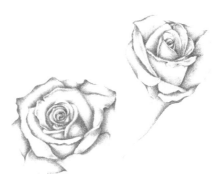

shaky paws and greedily gobbled up it's content. Heaven!

She needed more. Hissie grabbed another tin and another and another and finished them all so quickly she almost choked. What have I done? What came over me? It felt as if a big monster had invaded her tummy. It grew bigger and bigger by the second and soon she would explode. She had to get rid of it at once!

Hissie dragged herself over to the camellia shrub in her back garden and soon the deed was done, helped along by the vile smell of the nail varnish. Quickly, she buried the evidence in the moist soil. No harm done, she thought to herself.

On the way back to the house, she heard a strange noise emanating from the neighbour's garden. The noise turned into a groan that was followed by a big black and white lump that tried to squeeze itself through the garden fence.

'Won Ton, is that you? Where have you been?'

She was actually quite happy to see her brother again after her awful day. Won Ton was equally glad to hear his sister's voice after his traumatic experience.

'Hissie, give me a helping paw, please! I can't get this big bag through the fence.'

'First you get jammed in under the kitchen units and now you show up with a bag twice the size of yourself. Honestly, Won Ton, in my next life I'll happily do without a sibling!'

'Oh, His-Sis, please. Remember I promised to lose weight. I finally got hold of this new diet stuff I heard about. And you know, I lost my friend Met and put my life into mortal danger!' Won Ton was on the brink of tears again.

'Okay, okay, you've made your point,' Hissie replied, sensing a wave of pity and concern for her bro' as well as a sense of duty to sort things out. A shade of shame regarding her own behaviour came over her, as she put a wedge between the two fence panels, jumped over to the other side and together they managed to push the bag into their garden.

Won Ton was so thrilled to have made it that he gave Hissie a big hug. But what was that strange smell on her? A mixture of something foreign and acidic? Hmm. The two cats left the bag outside the larder and moved into the living room where they both collapsed onto the sofa. Having told each other all about their unforgettable days – though Hissie left out some of the details – they fell fast asleep, Won Ton feeling much better for having confessed about his antics at the bakery, Hissie less so for having concealed some of her behaviour. Exhausted, they fell asleep on the sofa and did not hear Aaron and Rebecca return home later that evening with the excitable dogs.

Aaron and Rebecca were quite amused to see the two cats curled up together – 'Like when they were kittens!' – in deep sleep. They also noticed Hissie's messy paws and the big bag of diet food.

Something was up!

CHAPTER NINE

A LONG JOURNEY

When Won Ton woke up the next morning Hissie had already left. He pictured the face of the angry bakery owner and thought about his theft of the cakes with a groan. All the other occupants of the house had gone too, which was something of mixed blessing. He was alone again, and really felt it. Thoughts about Methuselah engulfed him again. He had lost his life for him and feelings of guilt surged up in Won Ton like wildfire threatening to consume him. But then his newfound determination rose up in him again and he decided he did not want to dwell on yesterday's tragic events. He had to look forward and focus on his diet and exercise plan, otherwise his friend and guardian's death would have been in vain. With a big sigh he got up, stretched his aching limbs and ambled into the kitchen. Instinctively he moved towards the larder but was stopped by the big plastic sack, blocking its door. Won Ton had forgotten that they had placed it there the previous night. He fetched a bowl and cut open the bag. A whiff of something herby penetrated his nostrils. He poured a generous amount into the bowl – well, I can eat as much of this stuff as I like, he thought – and looked despairingly at the brown pellets. As he forced them down his throat some of them got stuck and he needed to wash them down with water. They certainly were as dry as sawdust and did not taste of anything much.

After his disappointing breakfast Won Ton went into the garden to start with his workout. Yesterday's humidity was still lingering and he was beginning to sweat already. Won Ton tried to remember what Mr Chickpea had recommended.

I think he said five minutes running and three minutes walking, thrice daily. So he went about running around the garden as fast as he could. With each stride, his belly moved uncomfortably from side to side. Won Ton was very worried that his legs might buckle under his weight. There he was, really pushing himself! But another round and his legs gave way.

Won Ton collapsed in a heap onto the moist lawn. He could not run another inch! Well, I'm dying of thirst and risk having a heart attack in this weather! he said to himself. After a while Won Ton dragged himself up and crawled back to the house. There he gulped down saucers of water and looked longingly towards the larder. But he stayed strong, thinking of Met and Mr Chickpea. It was so kind of him not to charge him for the Tom Trim. When he tried to settle down on the sofa he was so stiff he could hardly sit down. He switched on the TV groaning with pain.

A cookery programme. Won Ton wanted to change channels but became transfixed. In a trance, he watched the chef skilfully fry some pieces of chicken occasionally throwing them up in the air. And then he

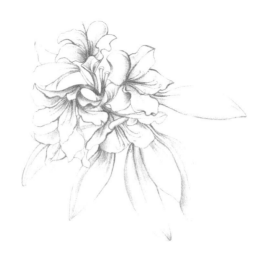

proceeded to empty a whole carton of cream over it
all. This was too much for him! Won Ton got up as
quickly as his state allowed and wobbled over to the
kitchen where he flew open the larder door. As he was
just about to reach for his treats, in his mind's eye he
saw Met gravely shaking his head. Full of remorse,
Won Ton went back to the living room, switched
off the TV and sat by the cat flap, where he waited
for Hissie's return. He wanted to tell her all about
his first day of becoming a new slim member of the

feline species. A feeling of pride spread through him.
I did it, I did not give in!' When he looked down on
himself, he thought his tummy looked a little flatter
already.

CHAPTER TEN

THE MATCH

A couple of months later it was a clear and cool autumn day. The trees looked beautiful wearing their colourful foliage and the air was imbued with a rich and earthy scent. Won Ton was in his local park enjoying the blue sky and the red and gold leaves of the trees around him. It was part of his weekly routine to come to the football pitch to support his team: Paw Eleven.

'Good pass, Rocky, that was wicked!' he yelled.

The long weeks of his new regime had been tough. Super tough. Won Ton had pushed himself to the limit with the exercises and religiously stuck to his diet. Only once did he relapse, munching throughout the night on whatever he could lay his paws on. But the next day he felt disgusted with himself and was back on track. Won Ton had lost quite a bit of weight and was getting so much fitter now, but he still had a long way to go to match the members of Paw Eleven. Perhaps today Won Ton would work up the courage to ask Rocky to teach him a few tricks.

'Goal! You are the best, Rocky!' he shouted.

They were leading by three goals to two and the rival team was beginning to look worried, as it was getting close to the end of the match. They started to run around like headless chickens, fouling anyone in their way. An especially nasty looking character jumped on top of Rambo (supposedly defence but more like offence) from behind and scratched his face ferociously. Blood was streaming down his handsome face while he was desperately trying to shake him off. They both fell onto the ground, but the nasty piece of work took the ball off Rambo and headed for goal. Won Ton's blood started to boil. What an injustice! This can't be tolerated! He darted towards the pitch and made for the offender. Won Ton leaped on top of him, just as he was about to kick the ball and flattened him into a cat pancake. Every one was a little bewildered, but

Bartok took advantage of the situation, ran towards the ball and scored the fourth goal. They had won the match! Won Ton jumped up in excitement leaving the nasty piece of work wriggling on the ground. All the Paw Eleven players came up to him hugging him and patting him on the back. Bartok and Rocky lifted Won Ton up on their shoulders and a hitherto unknown warmth spread through his body. I probably saved the match, he thought, feeling more than a little surprised himself. The defeated rival team left the pitch in frustration. Limping behind his fellow players was the nasty piece of work showing Won Ton his claws! Bartok and Rocky were still talking about the match long after it had stopped and the way Won Ton had saved the day. Won Ton was close to asking a player from Paw Eleven to show him how to dribble the ball when Rocky, the captain, approached Won Ton. Would he be interested in joining their team?

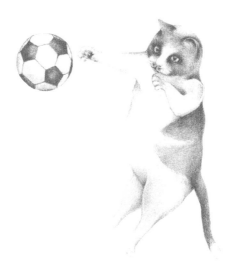

'We need somebody like you, somebody who shows compassion and courage!'

All the other players nodded in agreement. Won Ton felt himself blushing, but nobody seemed to notice. He was almost bursting with pride. This is the happiest day of my life, he thought as his teammates continued to cheer. He also noticed some sleek she cats eyeing him behind long lashes as they giggled behind their paws.

CHAPTER ELEVEN

BARTOK THE SAVIOUR

Hissie was sitting under the old oak tree at the bottom of the garden. The autumn sun was spreading its rays everywhere, making the leaves glow a pure gold. Whilst she was impatiently waiting for her beau memories of the last couple of months came flooding back.

Starvation, exhaustion, self-loathing and loneliness had governed her life then. Hissie did not want to dwell on this awful period any more. It was exactly

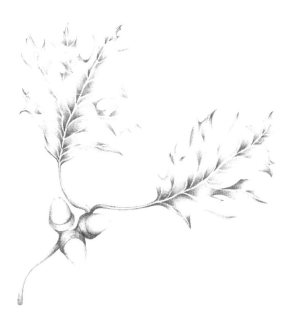

nine weeks and four days ago when they had first met. Hissie had been in the garden as usual, to hide the evidence of her predicament under the big, lush camellia shrub. She felt totally drained and guilty. Only the sour taste in her mouth and the burning in her throat indicated that she was still alive. It took a great effort to come out of her hiding place and walk back to the house on wobbly legs when Hissie felt somebody was watching her. Turning around, she could make out a black shape next to the fox den. Through narrowed eyes Hissie recognized the very handsome tomcat who had caught her eye when she was walking up the road with Barbie.

I hope, he did not see me earlier on, she thought to herself. Trying to look extra cool, she addressed him in her iciest voice. 'Excuse me, this is my garden and you are not welcome here,' she hissed at him, slightly higher pitched then usual.

'Okay, okay, Lovely, this is a friendly visit,' he replied with a dark, velvety voice.

'Well, you are trespassing. I want you to leave the premises immediately!' Hissie said.

But the gorgeous tom just smiled mildly and started walking towards her, fixing her with his beautiful blue eyes. Hissie was really annoyed now and her heart was drumming away in her chest. It beat faster and faster and her surroundings grew all blurry. The last thought she had was that her heart must explode any minute … then everything went dark around her.

She was floating in mid-air and a wonderful lightness took hold of her. Deep happiness flooded through her body. There was a very bright welcoming light and all Hissie wanted was to float towards it. She looked down and saw herself lying in the grass, being kissed by a very handsome looking cat.

Oh, this feeling of bliss and lightness … but the

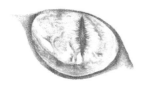 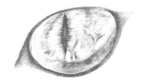

next thing she knew was that she felt dreadfully heavy. Somebody was sitting on top of her and trying to squash her chest. When she opened her eyes, two blurry, bright blue stars gradually moved into focus. They were in fact a pair of very worried looking eyes.

'Goodness, what a relief you are back! Oh, by the way, I am Bartok.'

What a beautiful voice, Hissie thought!

And so it was that love saved Hissie and she became more of what she was supposed to be, rather than less.

CHAPTER TWELVE

THE WEDDING

It was a beautiful spring day. The daffodils were swaying in a mild breeze, spreading their sweet scent through the air. All the other spring flowers were out and there was an explosion of colour in the back garden. Today it was full of creatures great and small and the anticipation was quite palpable.

Zooming up and down the ancient oak tree, Won Ton was adding the finishing touches to the decorations, attaching lanterns to the branches he had got to know so well. He was so excited and a little nervous. Today, he, Won Ton, would give his sister away in front of Rebecca and Aaron, Paw Eleven, as well as Methuselah's son and grandson Lamek and Ashur.

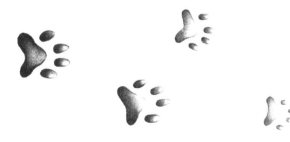

Jonathan, alias Mr Chickpea, and Aaron's friend with his two dogs Batsy and Lupinia had also turned up. Despite their difficult start, they had all come to get on well and the dogs had become quite attached to everybody in the household, to the point that were quite sad when they had to go back and live with their owner again.

Lamek had become a close friend too after taking over the reign of his father Methuselah. Today he and Rocky, the captain, had the special honour of performing the ceremony. Bartok was already by the oak tree, impatiently waiting for his bride to be.

When she appeared from the back door a gasp went through the assembly, followed by silence. Hissie's eyes were sparkling with happiness and her coat was ever so shiny. Being more curvaceous these days, she looked simply radiant. The bridal train and the beautiful white collar, covered in gemstones made her look like a star.

Won Ton rushed towards her, almost tripping over on the steps, and took his place by her side. They gave each other a wide nervous smile before making their way down the path.

Whilst walking slowly towards Bartok, thoughts of the past few months came up again for her. Her life had changed beyond recognition. Hissie, who had been suffering from malnutrition and associated medical problems, had come to terms with her past and made a full recovery. Thanks to Bartok's and Won Ton's love, support and understanding she was now able to enjoy food again. Very occasionally she would hear Barbie's shrieking voice in the back of her head: *You fat, clumsy, stupid mog!* Only last week Hissie had bumped into Jonathan who told her that Barbie was very unwell. Barbie's owner was one of his regular customers. Clearly looking upset, she had recently been to his shop to buy her soya milk and had told him, that Barbie was in hospital. She had found her unconscious on her bed, her pulse hardly perceptible. It was lucky they lived so close to the hospital! Now Barbie was on a drip and being tube fed. Hissie was not surprised. This was bound to happen eventually. She found herself feeling sorry for Barbie and re-solved to drop in and cheer her up. Won Ton had also had a tough few months to look back on. The most difficult times were those when he was by himself. What with Hissie being involved with Bartok, Rebecca and Aaron leading busy lives and Batsy and Lupin-ia gone, he felt pretty deserted sometimes, though he was developing new friendships with Lamek and Ashur.

Quite often he would find himself in front of the larder door, open it but then close it resolutely. Aided by regular visits to Mr Chickpea, who was such a great support, and weekly football practice, which always gave him a thrill, he was now the proud owner of a six-pack and was generally looking sleek! In keeping with his new, authentic self, Won Ton summoned the courage to tell Hissie how alone he occasionally felt and she came up with the idea to meet for a 'healer meal' once a month. The first time they went to their local Chinese restaurant and ordered baskets full of delicious little dumplings.

One dish took Won Ton by surprise: Fried little parcels filled with succulent meat and spices called *Wonton*! He just loved them and they became his absolute favourite. They even helped him to learn to like his own name. A sleek Siamese cat at the next table had wafted her paw in the air and told him Wonton means 'cloud' in Chinese. He no longer needed to feel like a 'one ton' heffalump! He was meant to be light after all! As he thought about his name he realized he had been created to enjoy delicious food – but only in moderation. He ate everything he fancied these days, but his portions were much less than before and he made sure he drank plenty of water and ate loads of fruit and vegetables because they made him feel good and look good. He found that if he ate a small amount of a variety of foods he was more than satisfied. If only I had figured this out before, I could have saved myself the trouble of the Tom Trim, he thought. But then I wouldn't have met Mr Chickpea and discovered my love of green tea, so all's well that ends well after all.

For Won Ton and Hissie, it was great fun just being with each other. They talked about their early time in the farmyard and what a lucky escape they had had when they were adopted by Rebecca and Aaron. Both of them spoke freely about their previous issues and were able to have a good laugh about it all now that they had overcome their problems. Sharing the same problem in different ways had brought them very close together.

Won Ton and Hissie were very fortunate cats indeed.

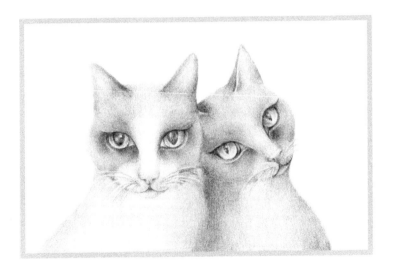

Lightning Source UK Ltd.
Milton Keynes UK
UKOW06f0952100116

266087UK00001B/8/P